The Weight-Loss Action Diary

A JOURNAL, WORKBOOK, AND MOTIVATOR FOR PERMANENT SLENDERNESS

by Mark Bricklin
Executive Editor of Prevention® Magazine

Rodale Press
Emmaus, Pa.

Copyright © 1979 by Rodale Press, Inc.

All rights reserved. No part of this publication may be reproduced or transmitted in any form or by any means, electronic or mechanical, including photocopy, recording, or any information storage and retrieval system without the written permission of the publisher.

Printed in the United States of America on recycled paper, containing a high percentage of de-inked fiber.

Library of Congress Cataloging in Publication Data

Bricklin, Mark.
  The weight-loss action diary.

  1. Reducing diets—Problems, exercises, etc.
2. Reducing—Problems, exercises, etc. I. Title.
RM222.2.B78   613.2′5′076   79-10591
ISBN 0-87857-264-3

2 4 6 8 10 9 7 5 3

Introduction

Inside you is the person you want to be. During the coming months, you are carefully and methodically going to sculpt this new you until it is fully revealed for all the world to see — **and for you to enjoy!**

You can't do a job like that overnight. Or with a careless kind of slap-dash attitude. It takes a certain amount of enthusiasm and stick-to-itiveness. That's where this *Weight-Loss Action Diary* comes in: When you finish reading *Lose Weight Naturally,* use this smaller book as a motivational aid and instructional guide. It's designed to be a kind of personal daily workshop at which the two of us can get together to discuss your progress and devise successful strategies to help keep you "chipping away" at your excess weight.

Slenderizing permanently is one of the most important things you could ever do to enhance your self-esteem and your health. Keeping this diary will help you focus your energy on the task before you, and make your weight-loss program considerably easier.

M.B.

DAY 1

Our goal is to lose weight permanently by changing our eating habits. Just losing weight, no matter how much or how fast we do it, is of no significance if we only regain it.

For that reason, the part of your diary which brings you into an action confrontation with your habits is of far greater importance than the mere recording of how much weight you lose each week.

In order to change anything, we first have to become aware of its present state. So let's take a look at your present eating habits. In fact, I strongly suggest not changing anything you habitually do for at least one or two days. Beginning too fast will only obscure your ingrained eating and activity habits and make it harder for you to see and understand them.

First, during the next 24 hours, I want you to record in this diary every occasion on which you put something into your mouth — whether it's a full-course dinner or just a cracker — even a glass of water. Record what you ate, how many servings you had, the time of day, where you were when you ate the food, and what you were doing just before you ate. Add any remarks you think worth noting. For example:

> **7:30 A.M.**—after arising, one cup of coffee with half-and-half, one English muffin with about 2 tbl. of cream cheese.

> **11:00 A.M.**—working at my desk when Susan came in with some cookies from her sister's wedding. She said they were delicious and told me to take some. I took one and she said to try the other kind, too, so I did.

Remember not to skip anything you eat, and to record second helpings.

What I Ate in the Last 24 Hours

DAY 1

What I Ate in the Last 24 Hours (continued)

(Day 1 continued next page)

DAY 1 *(continued)*

What I Ate in the Last 24 Hours (continued)

DAY 2

Continue to keep your eating and drinking diary for another day. Remember, the investment in thinking and observing you make at this early stage of your program will pay for itself many times over in the future by making it possible for you to improve your eating habits without having to rely on "willpower."

But during the second day, think a little more about each food contact you had. Record how you felt before, during, and after each time you ate or drank. For example:

> **Noon**—I was hungry because I skipped breakfast. For lunch I ordered a cheeseburger and a Tab. It came with potato chips which I also ate. I was still kind of hungry . . . maybe just dissatisfied, and thought since I didn't have breakfast, I could have a piece of cheesecake, which was small at this restaurant anyway. I ate it but it wasn't as good as I was told it would be . . . now, an hour later, I feel fairly bloated and dull.

It would be a very good idea to carry this diary with you and record your eating and impressions throughout the day. And remember — don't try to change your eating habits yet — wait until tomorrow!

What I Ate Today

(Day 2 continued next page)

DAY 2

(continued)

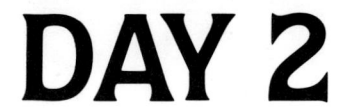

What I Ate Today (continued)

DAY 2

What I Ate Today (continued)

DAY 3

Look over the record of the past two days, and see if you notice any of the following patterns or tendencies. If you do, write down the details and any observations about this behavior that come to mind.

1. Eating when I am not really hungry

2. Eating more than I want because I can't seem to stop

DAY 3

3. Snacking a lot at a certain time of the day

4. Eating in places other than the dining room table or a restaurant

(Day 3 continued next page)

DAY 3 *(continued)*

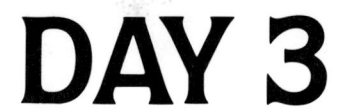

5. Eating because someone offered me food

6. Instances in which I regretted eating or when I felt unpleasantly full afterward

I currently weigh _____.

I want to weigh _____.

DAY 4

No amount of money can make me lose weight permanently, but if it could, I'd be willing to pay a maximum of (circle one):

    a. $3 a week;
    b. $5 a week;
    c. $8 a week;
    d. $10 a week.

Multiply the figure you checked by 260. Over a five-year period, that works out to a total of $_____.

Given the following alternatives, I would make these choices (put a check after the alternative you desire more):

    a. to be permanently slender
    b. to have in cash the amount of money I calculated above

    a. to be permanently slender
    b. never to have to go to the dentist again

    a. to be permanently slender
    b. to have a one-month paid vacation anywhere in the world

    a. to be permanently slender
    b. to be able to live six months longer than I would otherwise

    a. to be permanently slender
    b. to have a new wardrobe

In the above series of five choices, I chose "to be permanently slender" _____ times.

Am I willing to endure moderate pain (in the dentist's office) in order to be permanently slender? Yes _____ No _____

Am I willing to sacrifice some of life itself in order to live out my years as a more slender and energetic person? Yes _____ No _____

(Day 4 continued next page)

DAY 4

(continued)

I would rate my motivation to lose weight as:

    a. moderate
    b. high
    c. very high

I can think of the following reasons why I want to lose weight:

Right now, I feel that the most important of these reasons, to me personally, is:

DAY 5

If any of the following are true, write in your remarks.

Today, I found myself heading for the refrigerator, wanting to eat something, when I wasn't sure if I was really hungry. Here is how I handled it:

Today, when I felt thirsty, this is what I drank:

(Day 5 continued next page)

DAY 5

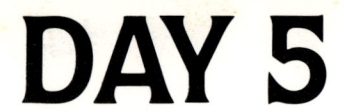

(continued)

Today, I began to change the following eating pattern:

Today, a family member made a comment to me about my weight-loss program. Here is how it made me feel inside, and what I said:

DAY 5

Of all the things that I did today, here is what made me feel the best whether or not it had anything to do with eating:

My observations about the above answer lead me to think that:

DAY 6

Eating properly is a kind of business, albeit a very personal one. And every well-run business needs to take inventory from time to time. Right now, it's time to take inventory in your kitchen. We'll list the findings right here in this diary; take it with you into the kitchen. First we'll look into the cabinets and pantry, then the refrigerator. It would be tiresome to list every last item, so skip things like spices and coffee that are basically noncaloric, and divide the rest very roughly into items which you feel are good foods for you to be eating, and foods which are high in calories but notably lacking in nutrition. Examples for the first category would be beans, spaghetti, and tuna fish; in the second category would be oils, sugar, cookies, cake mixes, etc. If you aren't sure which category a certain food fits into, forget it for the time being. You can also put a *plus* next to those foods you feel are especially good, such as whole wheat products.

Cabinets and Pantry

1. Foods That Seem to Be Well Worth Eating

DAY 6

2. Foods That Seem to Be Mostly Empty Calories

Refrigerator and Freezer

1. Foods That Seem to Be Well Worth Eating

(Day 6 continued next page)

DAY 6

(continued)

2. Foods That Seem to Be Mostly Empty Calories

If you had to rate your kitchen as it is currently stocked for the degree of help it's going to give your weight-reducing program, would you rate it (check one):

    a. excellent
    b. good
    c. fair
    d. fat city

How many of your favorite foods did you categorize as being essentially empty-calorie? _____

How many foods did you put *pluses* next to? _____

Which scored better, your pantry or refrigerator? _____

How many of the empty-calorie foods are purchased for other members of your family? _____

Are the empty-calorie foods segregated in areas where you don't stumble over them as you search for staples? Yes _____ No _____

DAY 6

How do you feel about throwing out foods which you don't really want to eat? Do you think it's immoral or wasteful?

I have trashed the following foods:

Quiz time: Put a pencil check next to foods you would consider appropriate for a weight-reducer to eat daily in substantial amounts:

      a. potatoes
      b. sweet potatoes
      c. raisins
      d. apple juice
      e. cantaloupe
      f. oatmeal
      g. potato salad
      h. eggs

Answers: In my opinion, at least, the following items deserve checks: *a, b, e, f, h.*

If you seem a little confused, consult *Lose Weight Naturally,* especially the chapters on "How Natural Foods Can Help You Lose Weight," and Appendix D, "Food Rating and Evaluation Guide."

DAY 7

Yesterday we took inventory in the kitchen. Today, let's look at food kept in other areas of the house — anywhere from the coffee table to the rec room. Include all alcoholic beverages kept around the house, even cases of beer stored in the garage. List all items. Put a *plus* next to foods you feel are well worth eating; a *minus* next to foods that you feel are empty-calorie foods, or inappropriate for a weight-reducer to be eating regularly.

Completion of Food Inventory

DAY 7

Which area seems to have the highest proportion of *minus*-type foods:

    a. pantry
    b. refrigerator
    c. other areas of house

How many units of the following items did you discover?

    a. bottles of soda (other than club) _____
    b. bottles or cans of beer _____
    c. bottles of wine _____
    d. bottles of liquor _____
    e. bowls of pretzels _____
    f. bowls of candy _____
    g. bowls of cookies _____
    h. bowls of nuts _____
    i. bowls of fresh fruit _____

Do you feel that, in general, the food you are keeping around the house is going to help or hinder your weight-loss program?

Are there any *minus*-scored items in your inventory which you think you might be inclined to eat less often if they were kept in a different part of the house? Give specifics.

(Day 7 continued next page)

DAY 7 *(continued)*

Is there any particular item you feel is especially likely to hinder your program? Any item you can't resist eating?

Is there any item or items you wish you didn't have in your house? What are they?

Can you think of any way to get rid of the above items — without eating them? If so, give specifics.

DAY 7

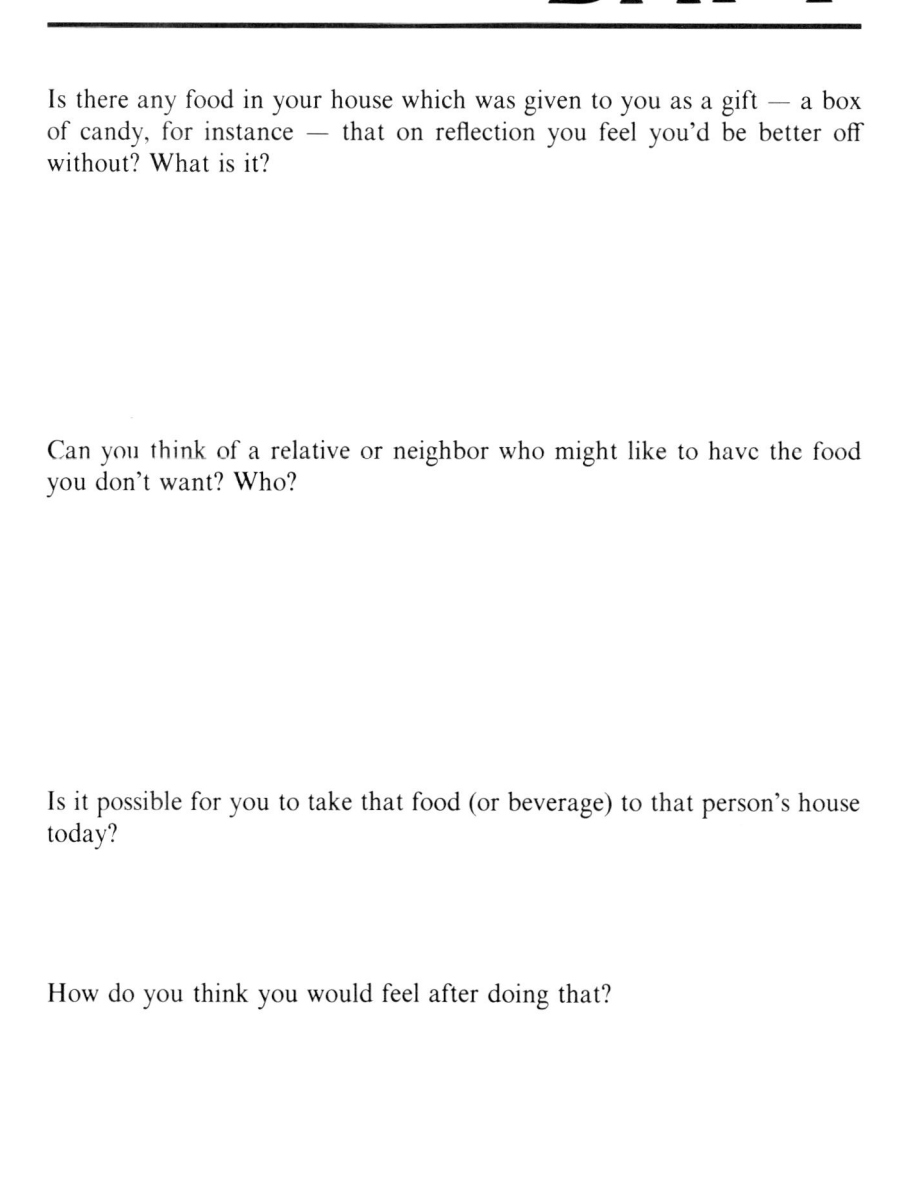

Is there any food in your house which was given to you as a gift — a box of candy, for instance — that on reflection you feel you'd be better off without? What is it?

Can you think of a relative or neighbor who might like to have the food you don't want? Who?

Is it possible for you to take that food (or beverage) to that person's house today?

How do you think you would feel after doing that?

DAY 8

Did you serve snacks to any guests who visited your house this week? If so, what were they?

Was that snack different from what you would have served two weeks ago? In what way?

Did you have a snack or snacks while watching TV during the last 24 hours? If so, what?

Was your choice of food different from what you would have chosen two weeks ago? How so?

DAY 8

Was your behavior when you got the impulse to eat while watching TV any different than it would have been before? If so, give details.

How did you feel when you finished your dinner today? (Check one.)
- *a.* unsatisfied
- *b.* satisfied
- *c.* more than satisfied

Was that feeling any different from how you typically felt after dinner two weeks ago? How so?

How did you feel 30 minutes after you ate? (Check one.)
- *a.* hungry
- *b.* satisfied
- *c.* stuffed

Was that feeling different from how you would typically feel after dinner in the past? How?

(Day 8 continued next page)

DAY 8

(continued)

What did you do today (or yesterday) immediately after eating dinner?

Was that activity different from what it typically would have been in the past? How?

Do you see any relationship between how much you eat at dinner, and what you do immediately after you decide you've had enough to eat?

DAY 9

Today I walked _____ blocks, not counting walking around the house or at work.

The most I walked this week was on _____, when I walked _____ blocks. That was because _____
_____.

I went up and down stairs today _____ times.

I did the following work around the house today:

I participated in the following sports or other physical activities away from the house today:

(Day 9 continued next page)

DAY 9

(continued)

Compared to my usual physical activities 20 years ago, my activities during the past year were (check one):

    a. much greater
    b. slightly greater
    c. about the same
    d. somewhat less
    e. much less

I think I would enjoy getting more exercise.

    a. true
    b. false

During the last week I took time to think about how I might increase my level of physical activity.

    a. true
    b. false

I have developed a plan for increasing my activity level.

    a. true
    b. false

This morning when I awoke, I felt:

DAY 10

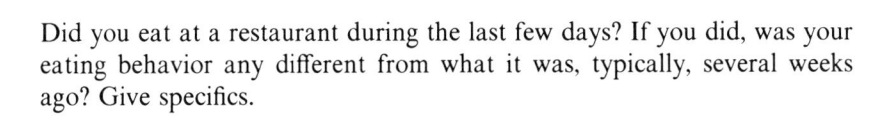

Did you eat at a restaurant during the last few days? If you did, was your eating behavior any different from what it was, typically, several weeks ago? Give specifics.

Have you thought of any new eating strategies for the next time you visit a restaurant? If so, what?

Have you eaten any foods this week that you have never eaten before, or haven't eaten in a long time? What were they?

(Day 10 continued next page)

DAY 10

(continued)

Put a check next to each beverage you drank during the last 24 hours. Also note how much of it you had, and how you felt before drinking it (such as thirsty, hot, cold, hungry, bored, etc.).

    a. coffee or tea
    b. soda
    c. beer
    d. wine
    e. liquor
    f. milk
    g. fruit juice
    h. water
    i. cocoa
    j. milkshake

How does your tap water taste to you?

If your tap water tastes unpleasant, could you possibly get drinking water from another source? Yes ____ No ____

Does something inside you rebel at the idea of spending money for water? Yes ____ No ____

Upon reflection, does it seem unreasonable to buy good drinking water to help you lose weight? Yes ____ No ____

Roughly speaking, beer and soda each have about 150 calories per bottle or can. How many calories did you get from these sources today? ____ calories.

How many calories from liquor, at about 100 calories per shot? ____ calories.

How would you describe the importance of the beverages you drink in terms of your eating problem?

    a. minor
    b. a factor
    c. major

DAY 11

It's been well over one week since you began your weight-reduction program, but you haven't been asked yet if you have lost any weight. Why do you think that is so? Give as many reasons as you can think of.

Look inside your refrigerator. Are the items closest to the door any different from what they were two weeks ago? Describe changes.

(Day 11 continued next page)

DAY 11
(continued)

The last time I had a glass of water was _____
ago. It tasted _____. After drinking it, I felt _____
_____.

I have a pair of shoes that are very comfortable to walk in.

    a. true
    b. false

Finding time to walk or exercise seems:

    a. difficult
    b. not easy, but possible
    c. easy

Walking makes me feel:

    a. fatigued
    b. pleasantly tired
    c. refreshed

I have thought about designing a walking route near my home that would give me 20 minutes or more of exercise daily.

    a. true
    b. false

I would like to get outside and walk more than I do at present.

    a. true
    b. false

During the last few days, I saw a person who was noticeably overweight, and I thought to myself:

DAY 12

Today, I felt good about the following eating behavior:

Today, I felt _____ about the following eating behavior:

During the last 10 days, I discovered that it was easier than I had expected to modify the following eating behavior:

It seems more difficult than I had expected to change the following eating behavior:

(Day 12 continued next page)

DAY 12

(continued)

It seems easier for me to carry through a behavioral change once I decide to try it than it is simply to try it the first time.

    a. true
    b. false

It is easier for me to make an effort to change my eating behavior than it is to carry out the new behavior successfully.

    a. true
    b. false

I consider myself the kind of person who likes to try something new.

    a. true
    b. false

Is your answer to the above question in agreement with your answer to the previous questions? In other words, if you feel that you like to try new things, have you been trying new patterns of eating?

    a. answers in agreement
    b. answers in conflict

Does it seem to you that changing and experimenting with your eating behavior could be a very interesting undertaking?

DAY 13

List as many hobbies or activities as you can that you used to enjoy but that you no longer engage in.

Do you think you would enjoy rekindling your interests in any of the above? Which ones?

(Day 13 continued next page)

DAY 13

(continued)

What hobbies or activities that you have never seriously engaged in would you like to try? Think of as many as you can and note them here.

Do you believe that, thanks to technology, modern man has more opportunity for leisure activities than the average working man or woman had 100 years ago? Yes ____ No ____

How much leisure time do **you** have?

Weekdays

Weekends

Are your answers to the above surprising in any way? Do you see any special significance in them?

DAY 13

What is your major leisure-time activity?

What did you typically do on pleasant-weather weekends when you were 20 to 25 years old?

What do you typically do now on good weekends?

List three activities you would really enjoy this weekend.
1.
2.
3.

DAY 14

How much do you weigh today? _____

How do you feel about that?

Have you surprised yourself in any way with your degree of adherence to your program? If so, give specifics.

Do you feel that during the last two weeks your impulses to eat have generally:

      a. increased
      b. stayed about the same
      c. diminished

Do you feel that the attention and effort you have given in the last two weeks to your weight-reduction program is in keeping with the intensity of your desire to lose weight?

      a. yes
      b. no

Do you agree with the statement of many physicians that the faster weight comes off, the faster it tends to go back on? Yes _____ No _____

DAY 14

How long have you been overweight? _____

Do you consider that one pound per week is an appropriate rate of weight loss? If not, how much would be appropriate?

If you were to lose one pound per week, how long would it take you to reach the weight you would like to be at permanently? _____

Does that length of time seem unreasonable? Yes ____ No ____

A handball champion, a man in his middle years, was asked by a magazine interviewer what he thought to be his greatest strength. "I can stick with it," he answered. "Twice in recent games I was behind 11 to 1, but I stuck with it, and my partner and I went on to win those games."

Think about that.

I feel I am the kind of person who can "stick with it" if the project is an important one.

      a. true
      b. false

DAY 15

The last time I went shopping I bought (check the appropriate items):

A	B
carrots	cookies
string beans	soda
potatoes	ice cream
mushrooms	lunch meats
beans	mayonnaise
broccoli	cake or cake mix
brussels sprouts	shelled nuts
corn	cocoa
whole wheat bread	jelly
rice	crackers
fish	candy
chicken	pie

My total from column A was _____ items.

My total from column B was _____ items.

My food purchases differ from what I would have bought a month ago in the following ways:

I feel that I am now shopping more wisely:

     a. true
     b. false

DAY 15

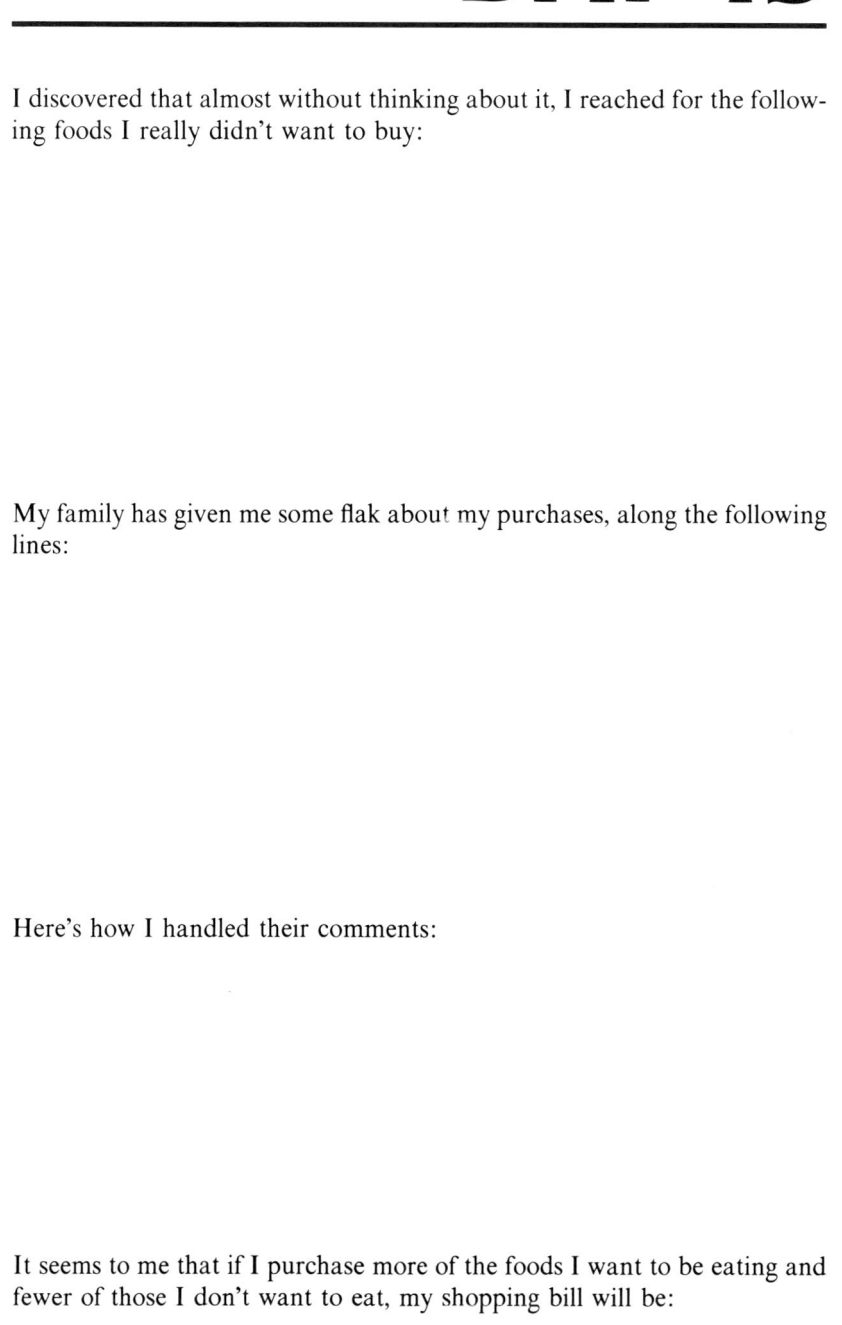

I discovered that almost without thinking about it, I reached for the following foods I really didn't want to buy:

My family has given me some flak about my purchases, along the following lines:

Here's how I handled their comments:

It seems to me that if I purchase more of the foods I want to be eating and fewer of those I don't want to eat, my shopping bill will be:

     a. higher
     b. lower

DAY 16

The last time I used the seven-minute-delay technique when I had the impulse to snack was:

Here's what happened:

While waiting the seven minutes, I did the following:

DAY 16

To reduce the temptation to clean up other people's plates by eating their leftovers after I finish my own dinner, I do the following:

The result has been:

During the last week or two, I tried this calorie-cutting modification of one of my favorite dishes:

(Day 16 continued next page)

DAY 16

(continued)

I've found that I can reduce the amount of oil I use in preparing meals in this way:

I've found that I can reduce the amount of butter I eat in the following way:

Today I drank water _____ times.

Today I ate the following foods which I think are high in fiber:

DAY 17

I believe I am most likely to snack (without being really hungry) when I (check one):

        a. watch TV
        b. read
        c. sew
        d. play records

I watch less TV now than I did last month.

        a. true
        b. false

I now spend more time doing something that does not seem to give rise to snacking impulses.

        a. true
        b. false

I've tried the following techniques to help keep myself motivated and following my program:

(Day 17 continued next page)

DAY 17

(continued)

The best technique so far seems to be:

I feel I would like to try the following motivational technique:

I have vividly imagined myself being at my ideal weight.

    a. true
    b. false

In those visions, I appeared to be (check one or more items):

    a. happy
    b. happier than I am now
    c. very attractive
    d. more active than I am now
    e. doing something I don't do now
    f. being admired by others
    g. more energetic than I am now

DAY 18

Compared to last month, my energy level now generally seems:

    a. higher
    b. about the same
    c. lower

I now seem to awake feeling:

    a. more refreshed
    b. about the same
    c. more tired

My feelings about this weight-loss program in general, so far, are:

I feel the most difficult thing about this program is:

(Day 18 continued next page)

DAY 18

(continued)

I think the following part of the program is simply wrong:

I've had the most success so far with this part of the program:

I feel I should probably spend more energy working on:

DAY 19

Some Thoughts to Think Upon:

If you went to a dance studio and asked to learn how to do a number of different dances, such as ballroom, disco, and square dancing, it would take you dozens of hours of practice until you had mastered the new steps. But then you'd be pretty well able to perform them without much conscious effort.

Moral: Don't expect to master the proper "steps" of eating wisely in different situations without putting in some solid hours of practice. But **do** expect these new steps to become much easier to perform after you've practiced them for a reasonable length of time. It's perfectly reasonable for you to feel awkward in carrying out your behavioral modification at this stage of the game. You'll continue to improve — even though you may not notice it — as long as you continue to practice.

* * *

The most difficult part of a long trip is usually getting to the airport.

* * *

Losing weight often makes a person look five years younger, and sometimes as much as ten years younger. It's do-it-yourself plastic surgery — with no scars.

* * *

Imagine meeting a friend you hadn't seen in years, a friend who'd always been noticeably overweight. But now she's slimmed down to her ideal weight. What would your first thought be on seeing her? What would you say? . . . Now imagine the same scene with the roles reversed.

* * *

Willpower never won anyone a mate. It never earned anyone a raise. It never painted a picture or built a house. It never saved a life. It never found a new path. Perseverance did.

DAY 20

What changes, if any, have you made in your typical breakfast during the last three weeks?

What changes have you made in your typical lunch?

What changes in your typical dinner?

DAY 20

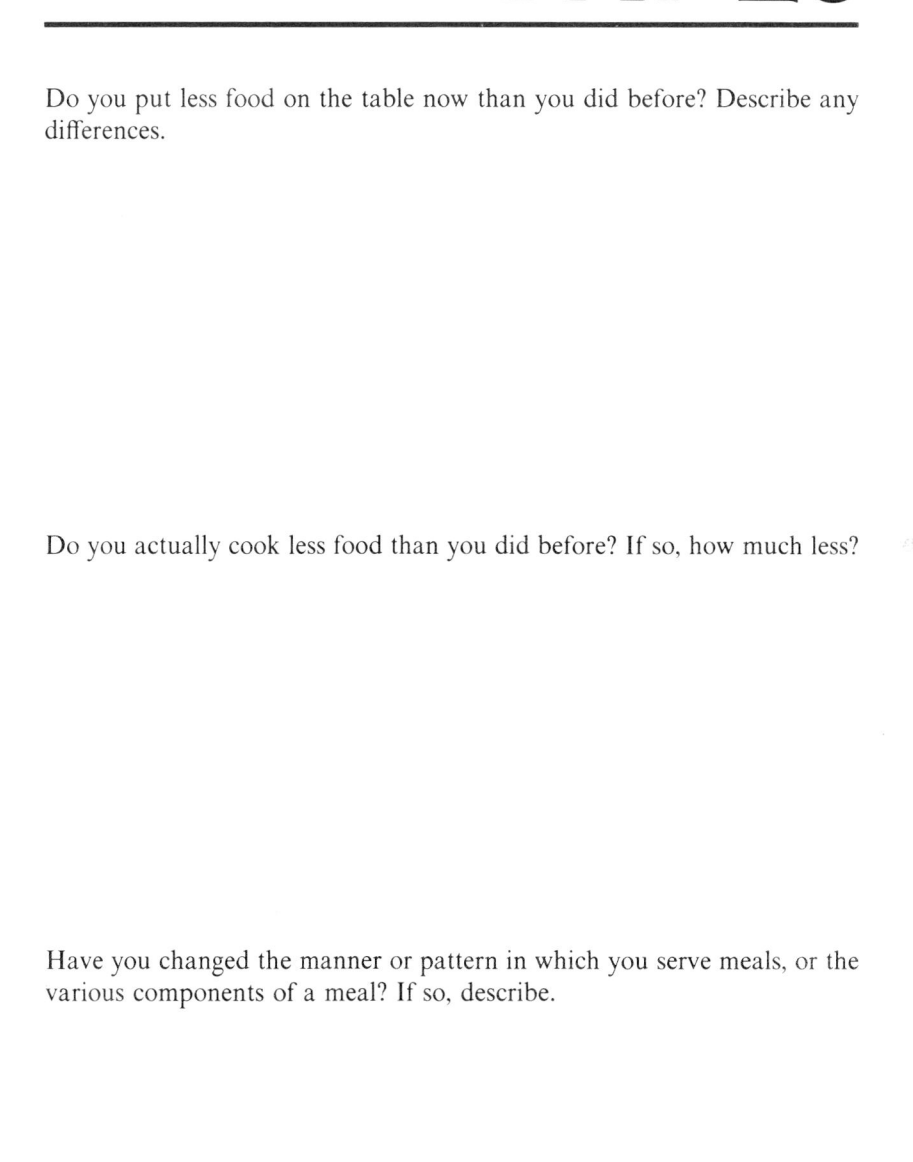

Do you put less food on the table now than you did before? Describe any differences.

Do you actually cook less food than you did before? If so, how much less?

Have you changed the manner or pattern in which you serve meals, or the various components of a meal? If so, describe.

(Day 20 continued next page)

DAY 20

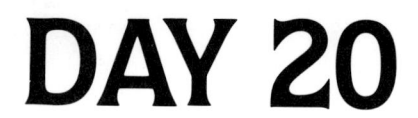

(continued)

Which of the following do you now use less of when preparing meals:

    a. oil
    b. mayonnaise
    c. tartar sauce
    d. sugar
    e. butter

Which item of those you checked above (if any) required the most ingenuity to reduce? Describe what you did to cut back.

Have you reduced the amount of fat in the meats you serve or eat? If so, describe how you accomplished that.

DAY 21

How much do you weigh? _____

How much weight have you lost during the past three weeks? _____

How do you feel about that loss?

       a. gratified
       b. not impressed
       c. frustrated
       d. discouraged

If the wisest doctor in the world told you that the faster you lose, the more likely it is that you'll regain weight, would you feel any different?

       a. better
       b. the same

Multiply the number of pounds you have lost by 30. The answer, in miles, is the distance you would have had to walk to shed as many pounds as you already have. You would have had to walk _____ miles.

Can you think of any examples of skills at which you are now fairly proficient, that were very difficult for you to learn — in the beginning? So difficult or frustrating that you sometimes thought you'd *never* learn? List as many as you can, from your school days to the present. Some possibilities: long division, swimming, golf, driving an automobile, etc.

(Day 21 continued next page)

DAY 21

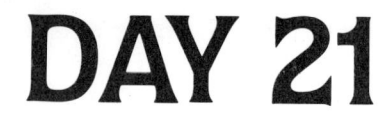

(continued)

Why do you think you were eventually able to master those skills?

    a. an intellectual breakthrough
    b. help from others
    c. perseverance

Sometime this evening, put yourself into a very relaxed state, using the technique described in the chapter on Super-Positive Thinking in the book *Lose Weight Naturally*. When you are fully relaxed, perhaps even in a self-hypnotic state, say something along these lines to yourself two or three times:

My goal is to be slender always. It doesn't matter whether it takes me three months, six months, nine months, or a year to reach that goal. If I stick with my program, I **will** become slender, inevitably. It's a good feeling to know that I'm progressing toward that goal. Important goals are never reached quickly. I feel good knowing that I'm persevering, and steadily working toward my goal.

DAY 22

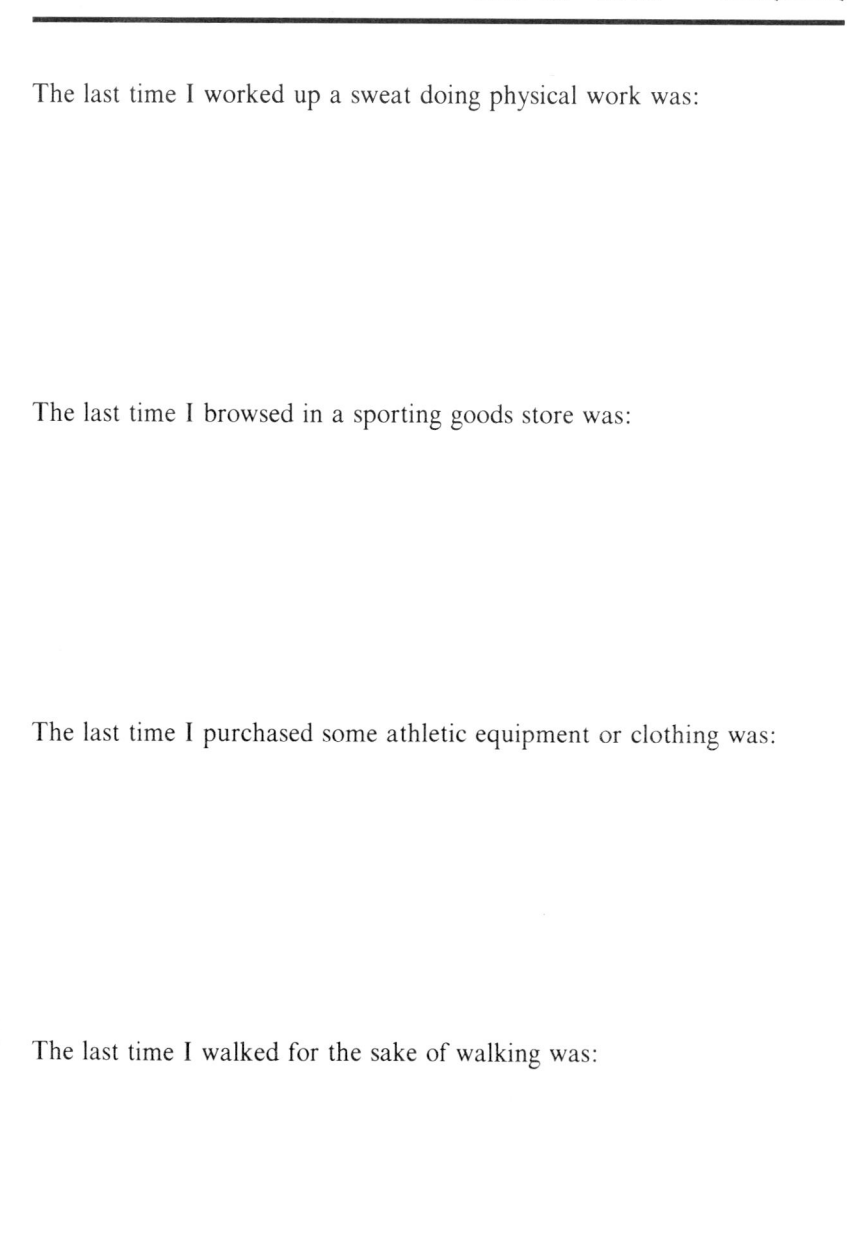

The last time I worked up a sweat doing physical work was:

The last time I browsed in a sporting goods store was:

The last time I purchased some athletic equipment or clothing was:

The last time I walked for the sake of walking was:

(Day 22 continued next page)

DAY 22 *(continued)*

I now own a pair of shoes that are very comfortable to walk in:
- *a.* true
- *b.* false

The following thought now comes into my head:

DAY 23

For breakfast this morning I had:

I believe that the following foods would be especially satisfying and filling for breakfast (check appropriate items):

    a. oatmeal
    b. cream of wheat
    c. bacon
    d. eggs and toast
    e. muffins and jam

Breakfast is (or could be):

    a. my favorite meal
    b. my most uninteresting meal

I have tried eating a larger breakfast than usual several days in a row, and I discovered that:

I would like to try eating a larger breakfast to see what effect it would have.

    a. true
    b. false

DAY 24

I have learned to enjoy all my eating in one special area of my home.

    a. true
    b. false

That area is:

I've discovered that doing that has this effect on my eating behavior:

I no longer eat while watching TV.

    a. true
    b. false

If I used to eat in bed, I don't any longer.

    a. true
    b. false

When I eat that is my only activity at the time.

    a. true
    b. false

DAY 25

During the last month, I have engaged in the following activities (check appropriate items):

    a. swimming
    b. tennis
    c. racquetball
    d. jogging
    e. yoga
    f. Tai-Chi
    g. archery
    h. hiking
    i. bowling
    j. skiing
    k. gardening
    l. dancing
    m. indoor exercise
    n. walking

I think I'd like to get involved in the following activity:

Here is how I would get started:

DAY 26

A Thought to Think Upon

You can become the person you want to be by simply pretending you **are** that person; by behaving like that person. If you want to be a person who weighs 110 pounds, and you now weigh 130 pounds, you will become that more slender person by eating as she does. And she is eating approximately 280 calories a day less than you. Or burning up that many calories in additional exercise. But you don't have to cut all 280 calories out of your diet at one time. You can cut out 125 calories a day the first month, 200 the second month, and 280 the third. At that caloric level, your weight will soon stabilize at 20 pounds below what it was when you began.

It's interesting to realize that it makes no difference if you currently weigh 100 pounds, 150 pounds, or even 250 pounds. If you eat like a person maintaining a weight of 110 pounds, you will inevitably become that person.

I would like to eat like a person weighing _____ pounds.

See the chapter "The New Math of Realistic Weight Loss" in *Lose Weight Naturally*.

DAY 27

During the last week, the following people offered me food when I really wasn't hungry, under these circumstances:

I ate the food _____ times.

Sometimes I think _____ is purposely offering me food in order to defeat my weight-loss program.

Here's how I've been handling that person:

Instances of having unwanted food offered to me occur mostly:
- *a.* at home
- *b.* at work
- *c.* at friends' homes

In general, I am getting better at handling these situations.
- *a.* true
- *b.* false

DAY 28

I have a certain place in my home where I can exercise.

    a. true
    b. false

I have a certain time that I exercise each day.

    a. true
    b. false

I take my dog for longer walks than I used to.

    a. true
    b. false

I feel very comfortable using an hour each day to do exactly what I want to do, without worrying about my job or family.

    a. true
    b. false

I have tried to increase the amount of time I can call my own.

    a. true
    b. false

Today I weigh _____ pounds.

A month ago I weighed _____ pounds.

DAY 29

A Cooking Tip: Make Meat Your Vegetable

Learn to regard meat, even poultry, as a kind of side dish or accompaniment to vegetables, instead of the other way around. Cut the meat into small pieces and slowly simmer with vegetables or grains. Let the flavors meld. A stew is a good place for melding. Use only half the usual amount of meat per person and add such vegetables as string beans, peas, carrots, onions, tomatoes, or lentils. Mix with grains such as millet, buckwheat, bulgur, or rice. Serve piping hot, topped with a generous dollop of plain yogurt. Let each diner add his own seasonings. Follow with a large tossed salad. Do not use cheese in a salad, except for possible sprinkling with Parmesan. If you serve bread with this meal, don't butter it. The bread can be dipped into the juices of the meat and vegetables.

I would like to try the following dish:

DAY 30

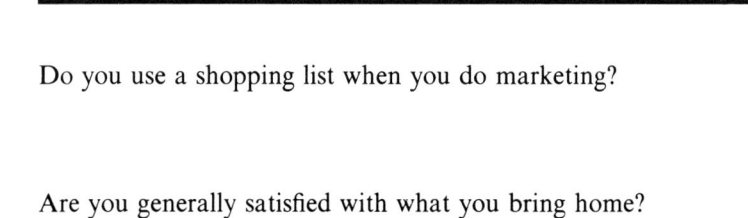

Do you use a shopping list when you do marketing?

Are you generally satisfied with what you bring home?

Do you know what your next dinner will consist of?

Have you tried any new recipes in the last month? How many? And how did they turn out?

DAY 30

Are you clearing the table faster now than you did a month ago?

Put a check next to the items you've eaten in the last week:

    plain yogurt
    bran
    fresh fruit
    carrots
    asparagus
    cabbage
    cantaloupe
    corn
    pie
    cookies
    ice cream
    brownies
    cake
    soda
    marshmallows
    whipped cream

DAY 31

Most people who become fatter as they grow older usually don't do so because they're eating more but because _____ .

If a person were going to a post office ten blocks away, that might be too far to walk, but what he could do in order to burn some fat is _____ .

If a person works on the tenth floor of an office building, that might be too far to walk, but what he could do is _____ .

I have the following ideas about how to increase my daily activity level:

DAY 32

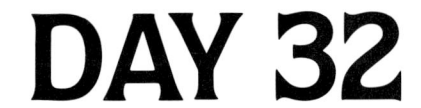

A popular magazine recently ran an article which told people "How to Lose 20 Pounds in 30 Days." What is your reaction to that headline?

Would your reaction have been different two months ago? How?

What would you say is a reasonable rate at which a person should lose weight?

What would you say is a reasonable rate for you, personally, to lose weight?

How do you feel about your progress so far?

DAY 33

How many recipes furnished in this weight-loss program have you tried? When did you try the last one?

Have you reread any chapters in *Lose Weight Naturally?*

Which chapters in the book were the most helpful?

DAY 33

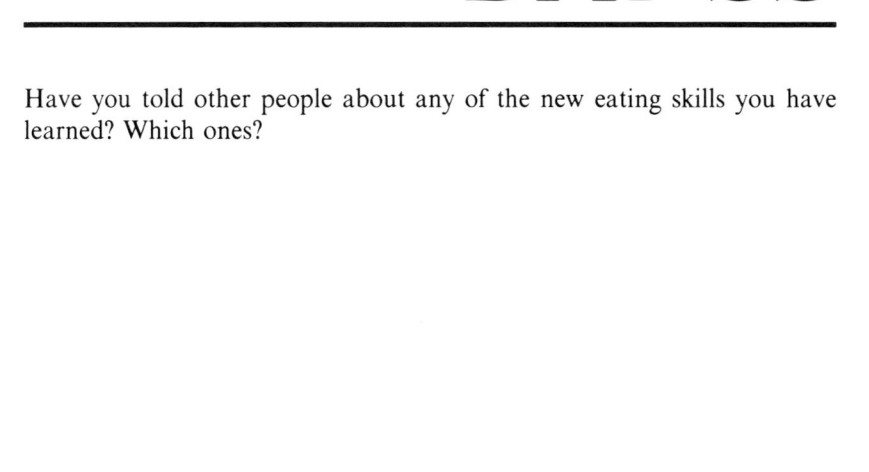

Have you told other people about any of the new eating skills you have learned? Which ones?

Is keeping this diary proving helpful to you? How?

DAY 34

During the last week or so, _____ offered me food when I wasn't really hungry, and I said _____.

Recently I accepted some food offered to me when I wasn't really hungry. Thinking back about that situation, I might have better handled it this way:

I think I handled one situation that came up recently quite well. Here's what happened:

DAY 35

I now weigh _____ pounds.

Five weeks ago I weighed _____ pounds.

I have lost _____ pounds, an average of _____ pounds per week.

Sticking with my weight-loss program seems to be getting slightly:

    a. harder
    b. easier

I have promised myself a reward if I lose a certain amount of weight over a period of at least several weeks.

    a. true
    b. false

That reward is:

I expect that I will earn that reward.

    a. true
    b. false

WEEK 6

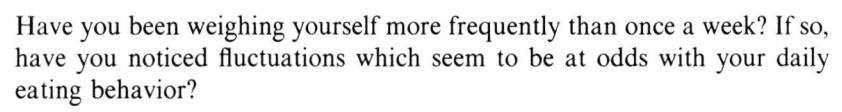

Have you been weighing yourself more frequently than once a week? If so, have you noticed fluctuations which seem to be at odds with your daily eating behavior?

      a. yes
      b. no

To what do you attribute these daily fluctuations?

What effect do they have on your mood or motivation?

Has your reaction to these fluctuations changed recently?

At the end of this week I weighed _____ pounds. So far I've lost _____ pounds.

WEEK 7

Deep down, I have a hard time getting over the feeling that walking when I don't have to is a waste of time.

    a. true
    b. false

I think that walking to get more exercise is one of the best things I can do for myself.

    a. true
    b. false

I answered "true" to both questions.

    a. true
    b. false

    If you checked the above question "true," you're in the same minor rut as many other people. To get out of it, read over the first two questions and your answers to them several times. Allow yourself to become very deeply relaxed and tell yourself that *anything* which improves your health or appearance is extremely important and worthwhile. Walking improves both your health and appearance and is therefore extremely important and worthwhile.

I now weigh _____ pounds.

WEEK 8

Check the situations in which you do not eat.

    a. watching TV
    b. reading
    c. watching movies
    d. when guests visit (except for meals)
    e. when there is leftover food on someone's plate
    f. when someone at work or at home passes around a snack
    g. when standing in front of the refrigerator
    h. while cooking
    i. while seated at the table waiting for others to finish eating

Add up the number of check marks. Give yourself half a point for those situations in which you still eat, but noticeably less than you did previously. If your score is six or more, you're doing very well indeed. If your score is less than five, turn to *Lose Weight Naturally,* and read the chapters "Why Am I Eating This?" "If You Really Want It, You Can Have It," and "Make It Easy on Yourself."

At the end of this week I weighed _____ pounds.

WEEK 9

Here are a few ideas and techniques for better eating habits from *Lose Weight Naturally* that I haven't tried yet:

Here are some areas or techniques I feel I should be devoting more attention to:

I feel that the skills and habits I am learning could be very valuable to me for the rest of my life.

      a. true
      b. false

If I could, I would like to share what I have learned with others who have an eating problem.

      a. true
      b. false

At the end of this week, I weighed _____ pounds.

WEEK 10

I have noticed the following "symptoms" of weight loss in myself (check all appropriate items):

    a. loose trousers or skirts
    b. belt buckles at a different notch
    c. underwear slips down
    d. rings seem looser
    f. shoes seem looser
    g. face seems thinner
    h. improvement of medical condition

I have noticed the following symptoms of eating a more natural diet:

    a. more energy
    b. less fatigue
    c. loss of excess weight
    d. improvement of bowel habits
    e. improvement of medical condition

At the end of this week, I now weigh _____ pounds.

WEEK 11

Has your change in eating habits led to similar changes in other members of your family? Give details.

Do you feel the weight-loss program you are following is better than others you've tried? Why?

If other weight-loss programs you tried were better, give details.
_____ (That's enough!)

I now weigh _____ pounds. I have lost a total of _____ pounds.

WEEK 12

How many people have asked you if you are "on a diet"?

How do you feel when you are asked that question?

Have you noticed that people seem extraordinarily perceptive of weight changes in others?

Do you have any thoughts about why that's so?

WEEK 12

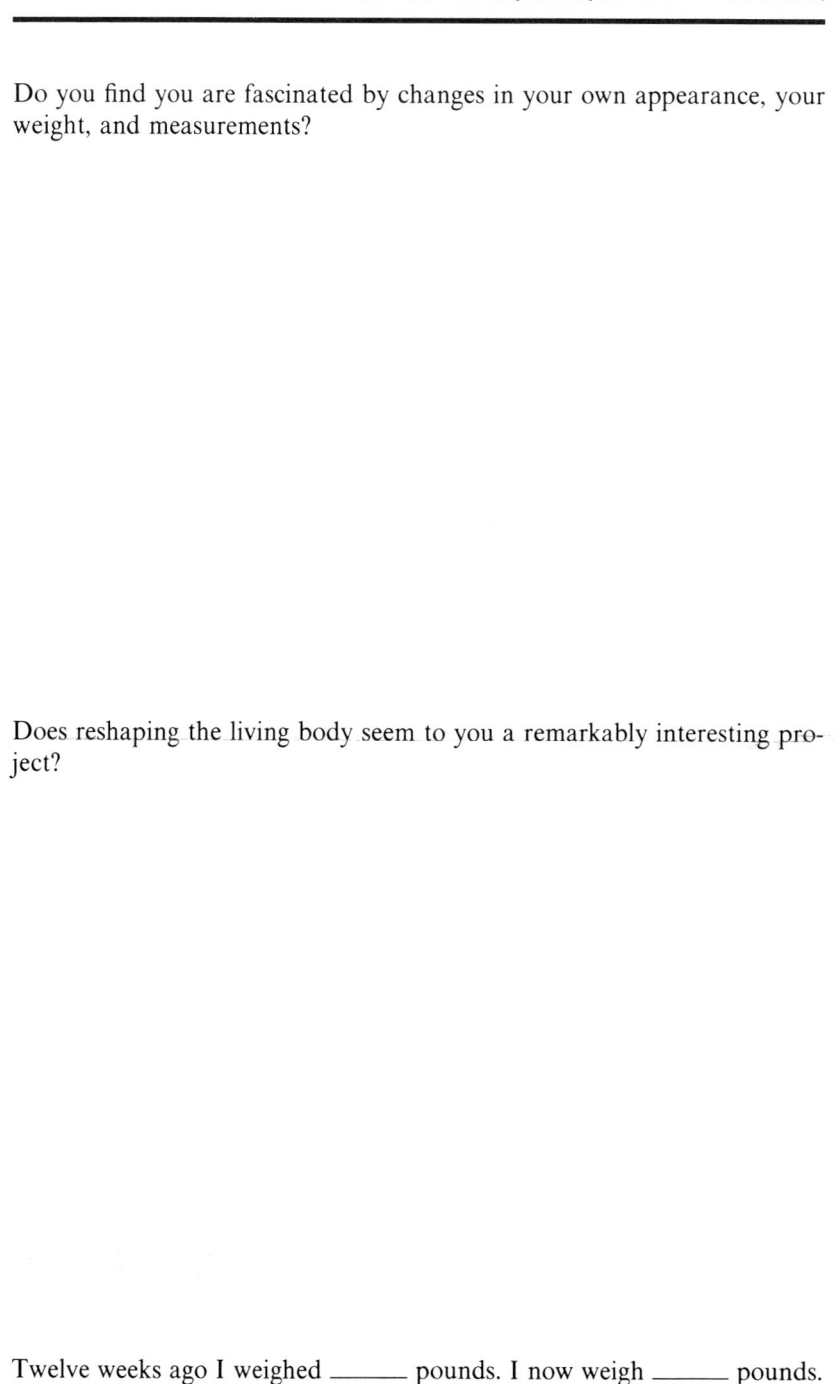

Do you find you are fascinated by changes in your own appearance, your weight, and measurements?

Does reshaping the living body seem to you a remarkably interesting project?

Twelve weeks ago I weighed _____ pounds. I now weigh _____ pounds.

WEEK 13

Have you recently put up any signs in your home to remind you of new behavior patterns you want to follow? What do they say?

If not, take time now to think of some signs you might make up and where you would post them. Write your ideas here:

I now weigh _____ pounds.

WEEK 14

Which of the following symptoms of weight loss have you noticed (check all appropriate items)?

- *a.* more energy
- *b.* less fatigue
- *c.* less need for sleep
- *d.* increased sense of pride
- *e.* people telling you you look better
- *f.* baggy pants or skirts
- *g.* purchase of clothing in smaller size
- *h.* feet less tired at end of day
- *i.* feet less puffy
- *j.* improvement of back problem
- *k.* walking faster
- *l.* face seems thinner
- *m.* arms seem thinner
- *n.* bones in hands more apparent
- *o.* thinking about wearing more youthful fashions
- *p.* disgusting self-righteous attitude towards people who eat too much

Today I weigh _____ pounds. So far, I have lost _____ pounds.

WEEK 15

Weight-Loss Math Review

How many pounds have you lost so far? _____

Multiply that number by 3,000 to find the equivalent in calories burned away. The answer is: _____

Multiply the number of pounds you've lost by 14. The answer is: _____

    The figure above represents the approximate number of calories you are no longer burning each day to move your body around and keep it metabolically serviced. In order to keep losing fat at a noticeable rate, it is necessary for you to have reduced your daily food intake by at least 200 calories more than that amount. In other words, as you lose weight, your rate of loss will tend to slow down unless you gradually eat smaller amounts of food or get increasing amounts of exercise. If your rate of weight loss has slowed down, that may be the problem. Keep in mind that as you become more slender, you are literally becoming a new person, and require significantly less food.

WEEK 16

Let the Big Ones Burn

No doubt you've seen exercise routines for slimmers published in popular magazines. They usually feature exercises to "firm up" the midsection, "shape up" the bust line, and so forth. However, except for a few minutes spent on stomach-muscle-tightening exercises, that kind of routine is not what you should be spending your time on, for two reasons.

First, such exercises give the promise of "spot reducing," which is a fiction. Fat reserves are taken from wherever the body decides to withdraw them, not from the area you exercise.

Second, the exercise which burns the most calories is that which involves the largest muscle groups, and *keeps them working gently for a long time.* Strenuous sit-ups, twists, stretches, and so forth are using only small muscle groups for short periods of time. *Neither pain nor fatigue are helpful in reducing.* The largest muscles are in the legs, buttocks, and back. Look at the following list of activities which involve these muscles for long periods of time and check those you do regularly. Put a plus next to those you would *like* to do:

    a. dancing
    b. roller-skating
    c. jogging
    d. walking
    e. Indoor Calorie-Burner exercises
    f. skiing
    g. bicycling
    h. tennis, handball, etc.
    i. _____

I now weigh _____ pounds.

WEEK 17

Are you able to eat a very large dinner or rich dessert occasionally without feeling guilty about it? Yes _____ No _____

How often do you have a dietary "blow-out"?

Regardless of your feelings, do you realize that occasional indulgences will not seriously interfere with your forward progress over the long haul?
    a. yes
    b. no

What effect, if any, do such indulgences have on your weekly weigh-ins?

What effect do they have on your desire for food during the next 24 hours?

I now weigh _____ pounds.

WEEK 18

At the end of this week, I weighed _____ pounds. I have now lost _____ pounds.

Do you lose noticeably more weight some weeks than others? Yes _____ No _____

    Think back to the longest trip you have taken in recent years. In the space below, write down every single instance in which your forward progress was interrupted. Note every instance from the time you left your door until you arrived at your hotel or other destination, including everything from red lights to circling an airport.

My Longest Trip

(Week 18 continued next page)

WEEK 18 *(continued)*

My Longest Trip (continued)

I eventually reached my destination.

      a. true
      b. false

WEEK 19

What is the longest distance you ever walked in your life?

What is the longest distance you have walked in the last week?

It would give me a pleasant sense of accomplishment if I could walk from _____ to _____.

Q & A

1. Which is more effective in reducing your waist measurement, doing 25 sit-ups or walking one mile?

2. Which has more effect on burning the excess weight around your chest, doing 50 push-ups or walking one mile?

3. Which has more effect on reducing your thighs, doing five deep knee bends with a 300-pound barbell on your back, or walking one mile?

Answers:
      1. Walking one mile.
      2. Walking one mile.
      3. Walking one mile.

Today I weigh _____ pounds.

WEEK 20

I seem to be eating less of the following items than I did six months ago (check appropriate items):

    a. oil
    b. butter
    c. cream
    d. mayonnaise
    e. sugar
    f. honey or syrup
    g. sour cream
    h. _____

Go back and put a second check next to items you feel you are now eating less of than you were about a month after beginning the program.

I have found certain techniques for reducing some of the above items in recipes, which I feel are worth sharing with others. They are:

I now weigh _____ pounds. I have lost a total of _____ pounds.

WEEK 21

Exercise: Now, More than Ever

Exercise may now be more important to your progress than it was a few months ago. If you have lost, say, 15 pounds, your body requires about 210 less calories a day to maintain its present weight. Therefore, even if you are eating 210 calories a day less than you were six months ago, you will not lose weight. To keep losing, you should now be eating 400 to 500 calories a day less than you were before beginning this program. That may not be easy, especially if you don't keep reminding yourself that you are a new person now, with different nutritional needs.

To help yourself at this point, take advantage of every possible opportunity for physical activity. That will ease some of the burden off your eating behavior, and help you keep losing. And the more exercise you get, the easier that exercise becomes.

I now weigh _____ pounds. I have lost _____ pounds.

WEEK 22

I have a tendency to skip meals.

    a. true
    b. false

The meal I most often skip is _____.

Skipping meals generally has the following effect on my eating behavior later in the day:

The later I eat dinner, the more I tend to eat for dinner.

    a. true
    b. false

If I know I am going to be really hungry for a snack in the late evening, I know what it will be.

    a. true
    b. false

It usually will be:

I now weigh _____ pounds.

WEEK 23

I now weigh _____ pounds. I've lost _____ pounds.

    Multiply the number of pounds you've lost by 30. That's the number of miles you would have had to walk in order to lose that much weight, if walking was all you were doing to reduce. Answer: I would have had to walk _____ miles.

To travel that far, I would have to walk from _____ _____ to _____.

Write three words describing your feelings about having lost the weight you have.

          a. _____
          b. _____
          c. _____

Of all the things you've done in the last six months which have caused you to feel good for more than a few moments, how high would you rank your satisfaction with your weight loss?

WEEK 24

If I have stairs in my house, I now use them more than I did before. Yes ____ No ____

> No? Reread the chapter "Exercise Can Do More for You than You Think" in *Lose Weight Naturally*.

If I drank more than one alcoholic beverage a day, I have changed my patterns of drinking in the last few months. Yes ____ No ____

> No? Reread "Undrink Yourself Thin."

I am often surprised — or discouraged — when I see what I have brought home from the market. Yes ____ No ____

> Yes? Reread "Shopping Wisely."

I'm still in the habit of cleaning up other people's plates. Yes ____ No ____

> Yes? Reread "Trash Your Fat!"

I now weigh _____ pounds. I have lost _____ pounds.

WEEK 25

I am somewhat disturbed by the fact that my weight loss has not occurred in the areas I most want to slim down.

      a. true
      b. false

If I am, I realize that these areas *will* slim down if I stick to my new eating program.

      a. true
      b. false

If I could have paid money to achieve my weight loss, it would have been worth $_____$ to me.

I realize that had I done that, I probably would have gained the weight back quickly, but that in learning new eating and exercise habits, I am now prepared to keep that weight off permanently. So what I have done is worth far more to me than the weight loss itself.

      a. true
      b. very true

Twenty-five weeks ago, I weighed _____. Today I weigh _____.

WEEK 26

I now weigh _____ pounds.

I have lost _____ pounds.

My average weekly weight loss has been _____ pounds.

I have reached my ideal weight. Yes ___ No ___

If not, and if I continue at the same rate of loss, I should reach the weight I want to live at in _____ weeks.

Two things I should pay the most attention to in the months ahead are _____.
and _____.

    While we have reached the end of this diary, I urge you to start one of your own for the future. Write down your feelings, your successes, and possible ways of overcoming your problems. Reread Lose Weight Naturally; *it will help a lot. And remember that while there are obstacles in your path, as there are in everyone's, there are no barriers. The skills you have mastered will enable you to meet every challenge, and to enjoy your more slender, more vigorous self for the rest of your life.*